CIALIS MEN'S USAGE MANUAL

Nicolas Petersson

Copyright © 2024 by [Nicolas Petersson]

All rights reserved.

Table of Contents

Cialis (Tadalafil) 1

Forms and Administration 1

Side Effects and Risks 1

Findings from One Study 4

Results from a Second Study 4

Cialis for Benign Prostatic Hyperplasia (BPH) 5

Effectiveness in Treating BPH 6

Cialis for Erectile Dysfunction (ED) 7

Effectiveness in Treating ED 8

Cialis for ED and BPH 9

Evaluating ED Symptoms 11

Off-Label Uses for Cialis 11

Cialis for Ureteral Stones 12

Cialis Dosage 13

Dosage for Benign Prostatic Hyperplasia (BPH) 14

Mild Side Effects 16

Blood Pressure Changes 20

How to Minimize Cialis Side Effects 23

Available Erectile Dysfunction Medications 24

Costs of Erectile Dysfunction Medications 25

Effectiveness of ED Medications 26

Onset of Action for ED Medications 26

Proper Use of ED Medications 27
Duration of Action for ED Medications 28
Cialis and Nitrates 29
Cialis and Alpha-Blockers 30

Cialis (Tadalafil)

Cialis is a prescription oral tablet used to treat erectile dysfunction (ED) and benign prostatic hyperplasia (BPH). Its active ingredient is tadalafil.

Forms and Administration
Cialis and Viagra are both available as swallow able tablets. Cialis can be taken daily or as needed for sexual activity, while Viagra is typically used only as needed.

Side Effects and Risks
Both Cialis and Viagra are designed to address ED, which means they can produce similar side effects, along with some unique ones. Below are examples of these side effects.

The following are some of the most common mild side effects associated with Cialis, Viagra, or both medications when taken separately:

Possible with Cialis:

- Pain in the arms or legs

- Heartburn

Possible with Viagra:

- Abnormal vision

Possible with both Cialis and Viagra:

- Headache

- Flushing

- Stuffy nose

- Back pain

- Muscle pain

- Nausea

- Dizziness

- Rash

Serious Side Effects

The following are examples of serious side effects that may occur with Cialis and Viagra when taken individually:

- Prolonged erection (lasting more than 4 hours)

- Loss of vision

- Changes in hearing, such as difficulty hearing or ringing in the ears

- Allergic reactions

- Fluctuations in blood pressure

Cialis and Viagra are both FDA-approved treatments for erectile dysfunction (ED), but they have different approved uses.

Clinical studies have directly compared the effectiveness of Cialis and Viagra in treating ED.

Findings from One Study
In one study, participants were divided into two groups: one group took Cialis either daily or as needed, while the other group used Viagra as needed. The results indicated that those in the Cialis group experienced greater improvements in sexual confidence compared to those taking Viagra. Additionally, the Cialis group expressed less concern about the duration of their erections, likely due to Cialis's longer-lasting effects.

Results from a Second Study
Another study involved participants taking either Cialis or Viagra as needed for four weeks, followed by a switch to the other medication for an additional four weeks. At the end of the study, participants indicated their preferred medication. The findings revealed that more than twice as

many individuals favored Cialis over Viagra, primarily because of its longer duration of action. The study also assessed the effectiveness of both medications using the International Index of Erectile Function (IIEF) survey, where higher scores indicated improved erectile function and reduced ED symptoms.

Cialis for Benign Prostatic Hyperplasia (BPH)
Cialis is also FDA-approved for treating symptoms of benign prostatic hyperplasia (BPH), a condition that can develop in aging males. BPH occurs when the prostate gland enlarges, leading to pressure on the urethra and resulting in symptoms such as:

- Frequent urination, especially at night

- Difficulty urinating

- Weak urine stream

- Inability to urinate

- Sensation of incomplete bladder emptying

For more information on BPH, please visit our men's health hub.

Effectiveness in Treating BPH
Clinical trials have demonstrated that Cialis effectively alleviates BPH symptoms. Researchers utilized the International Prostate Symptom Score (IPSS), a questionnaire designed to assess symptom improvement, including urinary urgency and weak urine stream. A higher IPSS score indicates more severe symptoms, while a lower score reflects fewer and less severe symptoms. The studies showed that participants taking Cialis experienced a more significant reduction in their IPSS scores compared to those on a placebo, indicating greater relief from BPH symptoms.

Cialis for Erectile Dysfunction (ED)

Cialis is FDA-approved specifically for the treatment of erectile dysfunction. ED is characterized by difficulty in achieving or maintaining an erection sufficient for sexual activity. Various factors can contribute to ED, including:

- Medical conditions (e.g., diabetes, high cholesterol)

- Nerve or blood flow issues

- Emotional factors (e.g., stress, anxiety, depression)

In some cases, addressing the underlying cause may alleviate ED, while other instances may require medication like Cialis.

For further information on ED, please refer to our men's health hub.

Effectiveness in Treating ED

Clinical trials have confirmed Cialis's effectiveness in treating ED. The drug's efficacy was evaluated using the IIEF survey, where higher scores indicated better erectile function and reduced symptoms. Participants completed the survey after four weeks of treatment.

One trial involved participants taking either Cialis or a placebo as needed for ED. Those who took Cialis showed significant improvements in their IIEF scores, indicating a reduction in ED symptoms. In contrast, those on a placebo either experienced no change or a slight decline in their scores.

Another trial assessed daily use of Cialis versus a placebo. Results indicated that participants taking Cialis had significantly improved IIEF scores, while those on a placebo showed minimal improvement.

Cialis for ED and BPH
Cialis is FDA-approved for the simultaneous treatment of both ED and BPH symptoms. While these conditions are distinct and typically arise from different causes, they can both affect aging males. For more details on ED and BPH, please refer to the sections above.

It is important to note that some BPH medications, such as dutasteride (Avodart), may lead to decreased libido and potentially contribute to ED. However, both ED and BPH are common in older men and are not necessarily interrelated.

Cialis has proven to be an effective treatment in clinical trials for individuals experiencing both erectile dysfunction (ED) and benign prostatic hyperplasia (BPH). The studies utilized two distinct questionnaires—one focused on ED symptoms and the other on BPH symptoms—to evaluate the medication's efficacy.

To gauge improvements in BPH, researchers employed the International Prostate Symptom Score (IPSS), a questionnaire designed to assess whether participants experienced relief from their BPH symptoms. These symptoms included urinary urgency (a sudden need to urinate), a weak urine stream, and difficulty urinating.

A higher IPSS score indicated more severe BPH symptoms, while a lower score signified fewer and less intense symptoms. The findings revealed that participants with both ED and BPH who took Cialis experienced a more significant reduction in their IPSS scores compared to those who received a placebo. This suggests that, on average, Cialis users reported a greater alleviation of BPH symptoms than those on placebo.

Evaluating ED Symptoms
For assessing improvements in ED symptoms, researchers utilized a portion of the International Index of Erectile Function (IIEF) survey. Participants with both ED and BPH completed the survey after four weeks. A higher IIEF score indicated better erectile function, reflecting an improvement in ED symptoms.

The results indicated that individuals taking Cialis experienced a more substantial increase in their IIEF scores compared to those on a placebo. This implies that Cialis users generally achieved better erectile function than those who received a placebo.

Off-Label Uses for Cialis

Beyond its approved indications, Cialis may also be prescribed off-label for various other conditions. Off-label use refers to the practice of prescribing a medication for a purpose not officially approved by regulatory authorities. One example of an off-label use for Cialis is in the treatment of ureteral stones.

Cialis for Ureteral Stones

While Cialis is not FDA-approved for treating ureteral stones (a type of kidney stone), it may be prescribed off-label for this condition. A clinical trial compared the effectiveness of Cialis with tamsulosin (Flomax), a medication commonly used for ureteral stones. The study found that a higher number of participants taking Cialis were able to pass their stones compared to those taking tamsulosin.

Ureteral stones typically originate as kidney stones before moving into the ureter, the tube that carries urine from the kidney to the bladder. Cialis may facilitate the passage of ureteral stones by relaxing the muscles of the ureter, thereby widening it and making it easier to pass the stones.

Cialis Dosage

The dosage of Cialis prescribed by your doctor will depend on several factors, including:

- The type and severity of the condition being treated

- Your age

- Any other medical conditions you may have

- The frequency of Cialis use

Typically, your doctor will start you on a low dose and adjust it over time to find the optimal amount for you. The goal is to prescribe the smallest effective dose.

For individuals with certain conditions, such as kidney or liver issues, a lower starting dose may be recommended to avoid exacerbating these conditions.

The following information outlines commonly used or recommended dosages, but it is essential to follow your doctor's specific instructions.

Forms and Strengths of Cialis: 2.5 mg, 5 mg, 10 mg, 20 mg

Cialis is available as an oral tablet in four strengths: 2.5 mg, 5 mg, 10 mg, and 20 mg.

Dosage for Benign Prostatic Hyperplasia (BPH)
For BPH symptoms, the recommended dosage of Cialis is 5 mg once daily, taken at approximately the same time each day. In some cases, your doctor may prescribe 5 mg of Cialis daily in conjunction

with finasteride (Proscar) for BPH treatment, typically for a duration of up to 26 weeks.

Dosage for Erectile Dysfunction (ED)

Here's an overview of Cialis dosages for ED:

If your doctor advises taking Cialis only as needed for ED, the usual starting dosage is 10 mg before sexual activity. If this dosage is too effective, your doctor may reduce it to 5 mg. Conversely, if the 10 mg dose is insufficient, your doctor may increase it to 20 mg, which is the maximum daily dose. Cialis should not be taken more than once a day, as it can remain effective for up to 36 hours after administration.

Cialis Taken Once Daily

Cialis can also be prescribed for daily use to treat ED, starting at a dosage of 2.5 mg per day. If this dose is not effective, your doctor may increase it to 5 mg per day. When taking Cialis daily, it should be taken at the same time each day, and there is no need to take it before sexual activity unless specifically instructed by your doctor

Cialis may lead to both mild and serious side effects. Below are some of the most common side effects associated with Cialis, though this list is not exhaustive.

For further information regarding potential side effects, consult your doctor or pharmacist. They can provide guidance on managing any side effects that may be troubling or concerning.

The Food and Drug Administration (FDA) monitors side effects of approved medications. If you wish to report a side effect related to Cialis, you can do so through MedWatch.

Mild Side Effects

Mild side effects of Cialis may include:

- Headache

- Heartburn

- Back pain

- Muscle pain

- Nasal congestion

- Flushing

- Pain in the arms or legs

Most of these side effects typically resolve within a few days to a couple of weeks. However, if they worsen or persist, consult your doctor or pharmacist.

This is a partial list of mild side effects associated with Cialis. For additional mild side effects, please speak with your healthcare provider or refer to the prescribing information for Cialis.

Serious Side Effects

While serious side effects from Cialis are uncommon, they can occur. If you experience serious side effects, contact your doctor immediately. If you believe your symptoms are life-threatening, call 911.

Changes in hearing can be a serious side effect of Cialis, with symptoms that may include:

- Difficulty hearing

- Hearing loss

- Tinnitus (ringing in the ears)

- Dizziness

- Vision loss

Other serious side effects, detailed further in the "Side Effect Details" section, include:

- Allergic reactions

- Blood pressure fluctuations

- Prolonged erections (lasting more than 4 hours)

You may be curious about the frequency of certain side effects associated with this medication. Below are details on specific side effects that may arise from Cialis. For more information, refer to this article regarding the potential side effects of Cialis.

Allergic Reactions

As with many medications, some individuals may experience allergic reactions to Cialis. While allergic reactions were noted in clinical trials, the exact number of affected individuals was not specified.

Mild allergic reaction symptoms may include:

- Skin rash

- Itching

- Flushing

Severe allergic reactions are rare but possible and may involve conditions like Stevens-Johnson syndrome (a serious rash). Symptoms of a severe allergic reaction can include:

- Swelling under the skin, particularly in the eyelids, lips, hands, or feet

- Swelling of the tongue, mouth, or throat

- Difficulty breathing

- Severe rash with painful blisters

If you experience a severe allergic reaction to Cialis, contact your doctor immediately. If symptoms are life-threatening, call 911.

Blood Pressure Changes
Cialis may cause fluctuations in blood pressure, with low blood pressure being more common. However, high blood pressure can also occur.

A drop in blood pressure is more likely if Cialis is taken alongside other medications that lower blood pressure. Symptoms may include:

- Dizziness

- Blurred vision

- Fainting

If you experience these symptoms while taking Cialis, inform your doctor promptly. They will help identify the cause and recommend appropriate treatment.

Though rare, Cialis may also elevate blood pressure, particularly in individuals taking it daily for erectile dysfunction (ED). If you experience symptoms of high blood pressure, such as headaches or chest pain, notify your doctor immediately.

Back pain is a frequent side effect of Cialis, typically occurring 12 to 24 hours after taking the medication. It usually resolves within two days. If back pain persists or is bothersome, consult your doctor for possible relief strategies.

Heartburn

Heartburn is another common side effect of Cialis. If it becomes bothersome, speak with your doctor for treatment options.

Prolonged Erection

Cialis can cause a prolonged erection lasting more than 4 hours, which may lead to priapism—a painful condition requiring immediate medical attention to prevent permanent damage.

If you experience an erection lasting longer than 4 hours while using Cialis, seek medical help immediately.

How to Minimize Cialis Side Effects
To reduce the risk of side effects, take Cialis exactly as prescribed by your doctor, either daily at the same time or as needed. Avoid using other erectile dysfunction medications unless your doctor approves. Never exceed the prescribed dosage, as higher doses can increase the likelihood of side effects.

Limit alcohol consumption while taking Cialis, and discuss any other medications you are using with your doctor or pharmacist to identify potential interactions that could heighten side effect risks. If you have questions about avoiding specific side effects, consult your healthcare provider.

The primary obstacle in finding the most suitable erectile dysfunction (ED) medication for you may not be related to biochemistry, but rather to health insurance regulations. Many insurers impose limits on the number of pills you can receive each month.

Once you reach this limit, the out-of-pocket expense for each additional pill can be quite steep. "The main challenge in my practice is the cost," explains Dr. Liou. Collaborating with your doctor is essential to secure the medication you need at a price that fits your budget.

Available Erectile Dysfunction Medications

In addition to Viagra, several other ED medications are available in the United States, including avanafil (Stendra), tadalafil (Cialis), and vardenafil (Levitra). These medications enhance blood flow to the penis, enabling an erection sufficient for initiating and completing sexual intercourse when combined with sexual stimulation. There is also a fast-dissolving version of Levitra, known as Staxyn, which is placed under the tongue.

Cialis is unique in that it is FDA-approved for daily use at doses of 2.5 or 5 milligrams. This can facilitate on-demand erections and may also alleviate urinary issues, such as difficulty starting urination, associated with an enlarged prostate.

Costs of Erectile Dysfunction Medications
The cost of ED medication can vary significantly based on pharmacy pricing, prescription co-pays, and your health insurance coverage. Even with private insurance, you may be restricted to four doses per month. Here are some strategies to help manage costs:

-Compare Prices: Pharmacy prices can differ, so it's worth shopping around. Online tools like www.goodrx.com can assist in comparing prices.

-Consider Pill Splitting: Discuss with your doctor the possibility of obtaining higher-dose pills that you can split to save money.

-Look into Manufacturer Discounts: Some manufacturers offer programs that provide a limited supply of medications not covered by your insurance.

Effectiveness of ED Medications
ED medications are effective in producing an erection sufficient for intercourse in approximately 70% of men. However, individual responses can vary widely. Men with nerve or artery damage due to conditions like prostate surgery, diabetes, or cardiovascular disease may not respond as effectively to these drugs. "There are some men for whom none of these medications work," Dr. Liou notes.

Onset of Action for ED Medications
The time it takes for these medications to start working can range from 15 to 60 minutes. It's important to note that neither Viagra nor Levitra

will be effective if taken after a meal, as this can hinder absorption. In contrast, Cialis and Stendra are not affected by food. The onset time is crucial for planning sexual activity, with Stendra and daily-use Cialis being the most suitable for on-demand use, while the others require more forethought.

Proper Use of ED Medications
Dr. Liou mentions that some men come to him after receiving prescriptions from their primary care doctors, claiming the medication is ineffective. Often, this is due to improper use. "The biggest misconception is that these drugs act as an on/off switch for erections," he explains. The medications require sexual stimulation to work effectively. "During that time, you should be with your partner and engage in foreplay," Dr. Liou advises. "Don't take the medication, then do

chores, and expect to be ready for intimacy later; it doesn't work that way."

Duration of Action for ED Medications

ED medications metabolize at different rates, with effects lasting anywhere from four hours to over a day (particularly for higher doses of Cialis). Each dose should be adequate for a complete cycle of intercourse, from erection to climax.

The following is a list of medications that may interact with Cialis. Please note that this list is not exhaustive.

Before starting Cialis, it's important to consult with your doctor and pharmacist. Make sure to inform them about all prescription and over-the-counter medications you are currently taking, as well as any vitamins, herbs, and supplements. Providing this information can help prevent potential drug interactions.

Cialis and Nitrates

Cialis should not be taken if you are on nitrate medications, which are often prescribed for chest pain. Combining nitrates with Cialis can lead to a significant drop in blood pressure.

Examples of nitrates include:

- Nitroglycerin

- Isosorbide mononitrate (Monoket)

- Isosorbide dinitrate (Isordil)

In certain situations, your doctor may prescribe a nitrate if you are experiencing chest pain and your life is at risk, provided it has been at least 48 hours since your last Cialis dose. After administering the nitrate, your doctor will likely monitor your blood pressure to ensure it remains at a safe level.

Cialis and Alpha-Blockers

Both Cialis and alpha-blockers can lower blood pressure, and using them together may result in an even greater decrease.

If you have benign prostatic hyperplasia (BPH) and are taking an alpha-blocker, you should avoid using Cialis. For those with erectile dysfunction (ED) who are on an alpha-blocker, your doctor may recommend a reduced dose of Cialis.

www.ingramcontent.com/pod-product-compliance
Lightning Source LLC
Chambersburg PA
CBHW070957220526
45471CB00007B/3066